Pocket Guide Top to Toe Examination

Anthony Whyte
Advanced Nurse Practitioner

INDEX

Assessment History

ASSESSESMENT
Presenting problem including use of **O** - Onset/Other people affected? **P** - Provocative/Palliative **Q** - Quality/Quantity **R** - Region/Radiation **S** - Severity/Symptoms other **T** - Timing/Treatment
Health beliefs incl. What does patient think is wrong?
Explores areas of particular relevance to presenting problem including "red flags"
Past medical history
Current health status
Current medication: OTC, Internet, Borrowed, Recreational, Understanding & Compliance
Allergies
Family history
Lifestyle (incl. smoking, alcohol, exercise, drug use)
Psychosocial history - home life, work, daily activities, outlook on life, coping mechanisms

The 7 Attributes of a Symptom

1. **Location**. Where is it? Does it radiate?

2. **Quality**. What is it like

3. **Quantity or Severity**.

   How bad is it? (If pain use scale 1-10)

4. **Timing**.

   When did (does) it start?   How long did (does) it last? How often did (does) it come?

5. **Setting in which it occurs**.

   I.e. environmental factors, activities, emotional, reactions etc

6. **Remitting or exacerbating factors?**

   Does anything make it better or worse?

7. **Associated manifestation.**

   Have you noticed anything else that accompanies it?

GENERAL SURVEY - Observe throughout contact.

[Some overlaps with Mental Status]

- **APPEARANCE** - health status, colour, stature, sexual development, weight, posture, dress, grooming, hygiene, odours
- **ACTIVITY** - gait, motor activity, expression, speech (voice – CN IX Glossopharyngeal & CN X Vagus)

MENTAL STATUS

- **Observe and interview to assess consciousness, thought processes, general coherence, interactions, mood and behaviour**
- **Orientation**
  Where are we (state) (country) (town) (hospital)   (floor) What is the (year) (season) (date) (day) (month)

THORAX AND LUNGS

Assess anteriorly then posteriorly with client sitting if possible. For posterior ask to cross arms over chest.

> **INSPECTION** - size, shape and symmetry; AP to lateral ratio (normal 1:2); & respiratory effort and type

> **PALPATION** - Note characteristics of underlying tissues. Expansion posteriorly and fremitus (6 sites anteriorly, 8 posteriorly).

> **PERCUSSION** – using side-to-side comparison (4 medial and 2 lateral sites both sides anterior, and 5 medial and 2 lateral sites both sides posterior) for resonance throughout. Measure diaphragmatic excursion on both sides posteriorly.

> **AUSCULTATION** - using diaphragm of stethoscope, compare sounds at same sites used for percussion. Note sound type (vesicular, bronchovesicular, bronchial), pitch, intensity, duration in

inspiration and expiration; and absence of adventitious sounds (crackles, wheezes, rubs).

Chest Exam

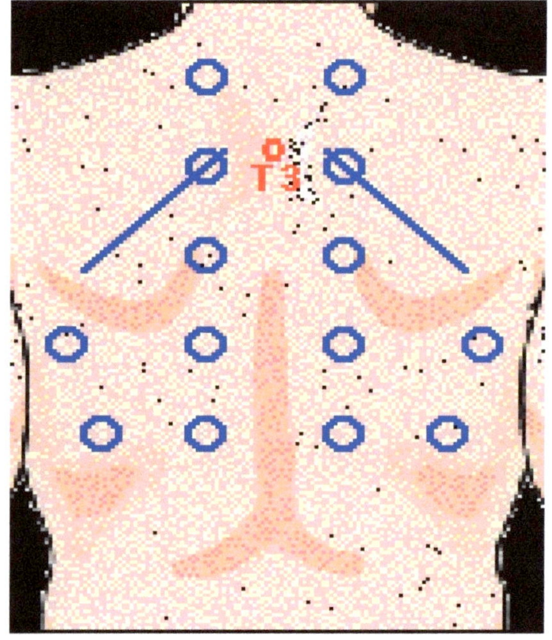

Posterior

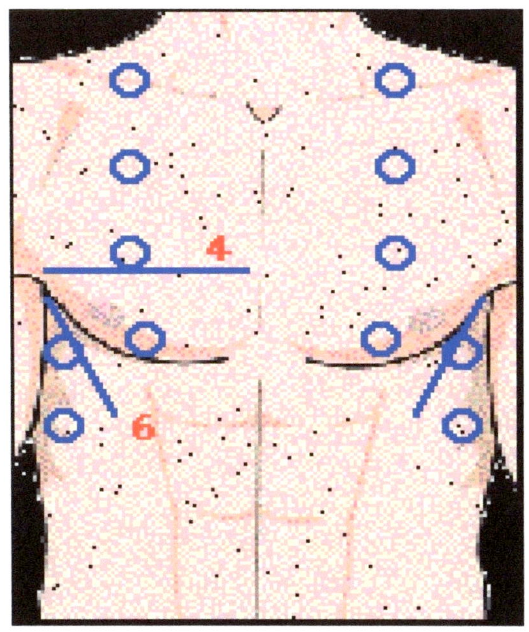

Anterior

CARDIOVASCULAR

- ➢ **INSPECTION** - using tangential light assess position of apical impulse. Note absence of lift and heaves.
- ➢ **PALPATION** – note absence of lifts, heaves and thrills. Identify location of apical impulse noting amplitude, diameter, duration awareness of special manoeuvre to illicit nature of apex beat (lay on left side).
- ➢ **AUSCULTATION** - listen with bell and diaphragm of stethoscope at right 2nd intercostal space (aortic), left 2nd interspace (pulmonary), left 3rd interspace, left 4th and 5th interspaces at lower left sterna border (tricuspid), and the apex (mitral area) at 5th left interspace 7-9cm from midsternal line. Note character of S1 and S2, presence or absence of splits, S3, S4, murmur, click, snap or rub.
- ➢ **SPECIAL MANOEUVRES** - Client rolls partly toward the left side - listen with bell at apical impulse (for mitral murmurs). With client sitting and leaning forward ask to

exhale and hold breath - listen with diaphragm along lower sternal border 3rd, 4th & 5th and at apex (aortic murmurs)

Cardiac Exam

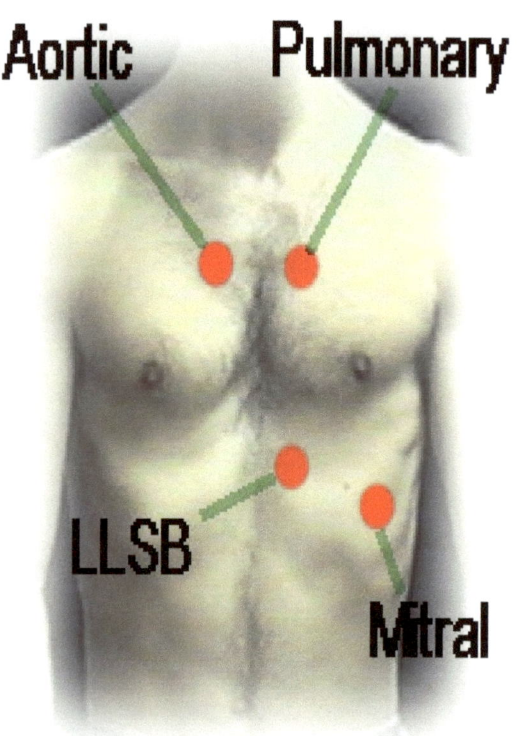

ABDOMEN

(Use techniques in different order than other systems).

- ➤ **INSPECTION** - using tangential light - shape, symmetry, contour, movement, umbilicus, and absence of scars or hernias
- ➤ **AUSCULTATION** - noting frequency and equality of bowel sounds in all 4 quadrants, absence of bruits from vessels (iliac and renal arteries and aorta)
- ➤ **PERCUSSION** - 4 quadrants for general tympany, gastric air bubble, and bladder. Measure liver span at right midclavicular line.

PALPATION

- ➢ **LIGHT** – over aorta noting pulsation and width, and then generally for absence of masses or tenderness.
- ➢ **DEEP, REBOUND** - for absence of masses and tenderness including rebound tenderness & Rovsing's sign if indecated
- ➢ **BIMANUAL ORGANS** (liver & spleen) – start below umbilicus noting absence of enlargement. (If palpable note size, consistency, irregularities, tenderness).
- ➢ **KIDNEYS** – bimanual palpation for size & tenderness consider testing for CVA tenderness indirectly, both sides.
- ➢ **INGUINAL** - lymph nodes horizontal and vertical. Note absence of hernias.

Abdominal Exam

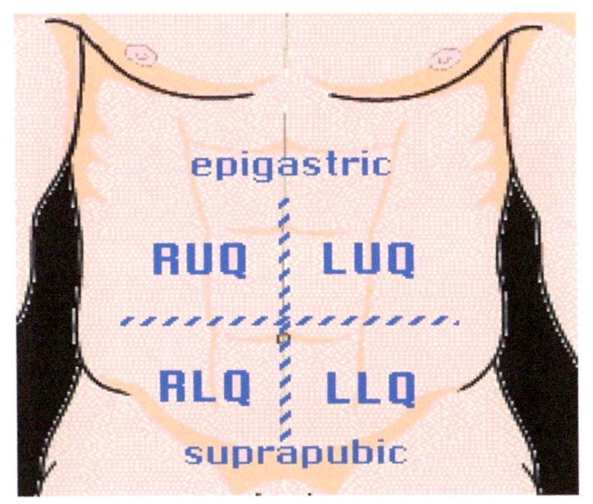

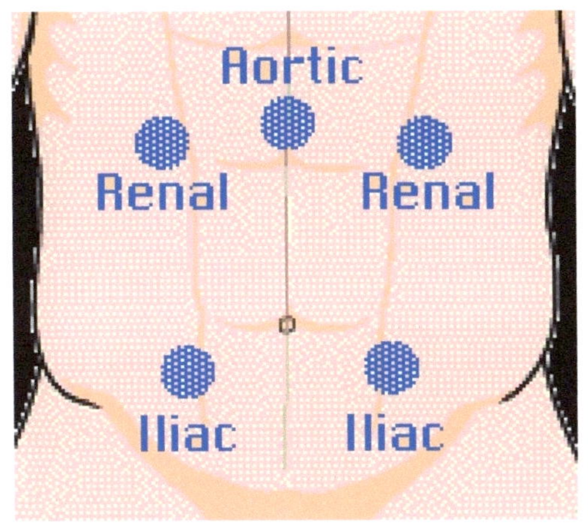

Genitalia & Rectal

Pelvic examination (involving inspection and palpation of the vagina, cervix and rectum and palpation of the uterus and adnexae)
Male and female external examinations and rectal examinations should be practiced in appropriate clinical situations.

Inspection and palpation of the external female genitalia includes the vulva, perineum and anus. Inspection and palpation of the male genitalia includes the penis, scrotum, testes, perineum, anus, inguinal canal and prostate during rectal exam.

SKIN

Inspect and palpate for colour, vascularity, temperature, texture, turgor, elasticity, moisture and absence of lesions. Assessment is integrated throughout examination.

- **HAIR** - colour, texture and distribution on head and body
- **NAILS** - colour, shape, angle (clubbing), beds, and capillary refill
- **HEAD** - Inspect and palpate skull and scalp parting hair and noting shape, contour, symmetry and absence of lesions
- **FACE** - Inspect and palpate for size, shape, symmetry, and notable characteristics.
- **FACIES** at rest and in movement (smile, frown, wrinkle forehead) (**CN VII Facial**)
- **JAW** - clench, open, side-to-side (**CN V Trigeminal**) and assess TMJ for tenderness, crepitus.

Ear, Nose Throat (ENT)

EYES

Inspect for placement and symmetry.

> **ACUITY** - using Snellen, or gross reading ability, and colour vision (**CN II Optic**)

> **VISUAL FIELDS** - by confrontation in 8 fields of both eyes (**CN II**)

> **EOMs** Note extraocular movements as being conjugate in 6 cardinal fields of gaze plus convergence and no more than 3 beats of nystagmus on lateral gaze (**CN III Oculomotor, CN IV Trochlear, CN VI Abducens**).

> **EXTERNAL** - inspect lashes, brows, lids, (**CN III, IV, VI**) lacrimal apparatus, sclerae, conjunctivae, irises, and corneas. Corneal reflex (**CN V & VII**) deferred in class.

> **PUPILS** - note size, shape, pupillary reaction to light, (direct and consensual) and accommodation (PERRLA) (**CN III, II**)

> **FUNDOSCOPY**-inspect red reflex, lens (opacity), optic disc and cup (colour and size), retinal blood vessels (AV ratio, size and crossings), background, macular area, and fovea (**CN II Optic**)

EARS

- **ACUITY** - audiometric measurements or whispers (**CN VIII Acoustic**)
- **WEBER**, **RINNE** using tuning fork (512Hz) to check for absence of abnormal lateralisation (Weber) and for normal finding of air conduction being greater than bone conduction (Rinne) (**CN VIII**) AC > BC
- **EXTERNAL** - inspect and palpate auricle, tragus and mastoid both ears
- **CANALS** -inspect externally and internally for shape, size and patency
- **EARDRUMS** - using auroscope, inspect tympanic membranes for landmarks (cone of light, umbo, long and short processes of malleus), colour, intactness and margins

NOSE

SENSE OF SMELL - assess patency then ability to identify odours such as vanilla and cloves one side at a time (CN I Olfactory)

- ➤ **EXTERNAL** - inspect for size, shape and symmetry
- ➤ **INTERNAL** - inspect internal septum, membranes, hydration and turbinates
- ➤ **SINUSES** - palpate frontal and maxillary areas for absence of tenderness

MOUTH

- ➢ **TASTE** – verbalise assessing posterior third of tongue bilaterally for bitter (**CN IX Glossopharyngeal)** and then anterior two thirds bilaterally for sweet, salty, sour and bitter **(CN VII**)
- ➢ **EXTERNAL** - lips for colour and shape
- ➢ **TEETH** - number, position and occlusion and gingiva
- ➢ **BUCCAL CAVITY** - inspect using tongue depressor noting palate rising on phonation, uvula midline (**CN IX & X**), palpate Stensen's (parotid) and Wharton's (submandibular) ducts using gloved finger. Gag reflex (**CN IX & X**)
- ➢ **TONGUE** - appearance, mobility, strength (**CN XII Hypoglossal**)
- ➢ **MUCOSA** - colour and character of mouth and throat, pharynx, pillars and tonsils

NECK

- ➢ **TRACHEA** - in midline (place finger between trachea and sternomastoid on both sides)
- ➢ **THYROID** - swallow (**CN IX & X**), locate isthmus and palpate lobes of gland from behind

LYMPH NODES

Palpate using pads of fingers and rolling motion noting whether or not nodes are palpable (If so note size, mobility, consistency, and absence of tenderness as well as temperature and colour of overlying skin).   [Inguinal nodes may be assessed after the abdominal examination]

> **HEAD** - occipital and pre and post auricular
> **JAW** - tonsillar, submandibular, and submental
> **CERVICAL** - superficial, posterior and deep
> **SUPRA CLAVICULAR**
> **AXILLARY** - anterior pectoral, posterior or subscapular, central and lateral
> **EPITROCHLEAR** - above elbow below medial biceps.

The 3-minute neurological examination

Designed to exclude sinister causes of headache including brain tumour and haemorrhage. The brief neurological examination is suitable for patients whose history suggests migraine or tension-type headaches.

Examination	Notes
Romberg's test	Patient falling with eyes closed.
Tandem gait test	Heel-to-toe walking
Walking on heels	
Drift of outstretched arms	Tests pyramidal tract.
Finger-nose test	Tests coordination.
Fine finger movements	Tests pyramidal and extrapyramidal tracts.
Hand tapping.	Cerebellar and brainstem disease.
Visual fields to confrontation	
Eye movements	
Face and tongue movements	
Fundoscopy	
Reflexes	

GP Notebook

The 12 Cranial Nerves

Cranial Nerve:	Major Functions:
I Olfactory	Smell
II Optic	vision
III Oculomotor	eyelid and eyeball movement
IV Trochlea	innervates superior oblique turns eye downward & laterally
V Trigeminal	chewing face & mouth touch & pain
VI Abducens	turns eye laterally
VII Facial	controls most facial expressions & secretion
VIII (auditory)	hearing equilibrium sensation Vestibulocochlear
IX Glossopharyngeal	tongue and pharynx.
X Vagus	senses aortic blood pressure slows heart rate stimulates digestive organs taste
XI Spinal Accessory	controls trapezius & sternocleidomastoid controls swallowing movements
XII Hypoglossal	controls tongue movements

Cranial Nerves

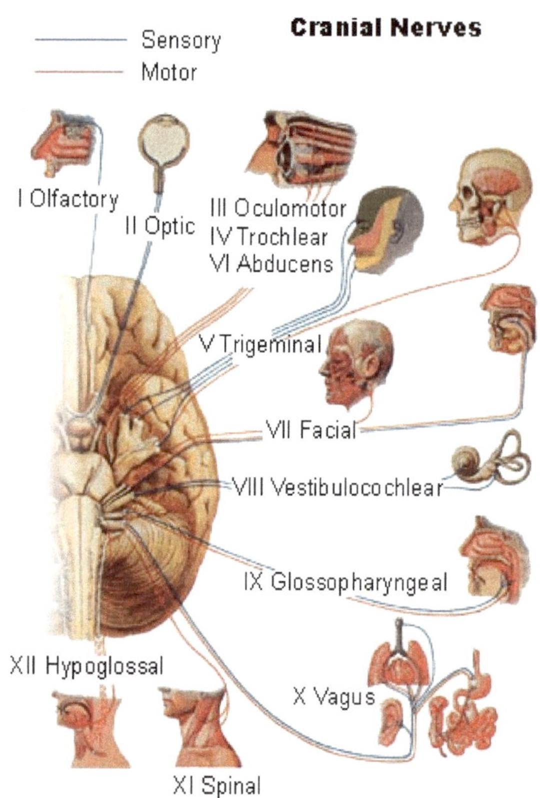

PERIPHERAL VASCULAR

- ➤ **INSPECT & PALPATE UPPER LIMBS** – for oedema, colour, vascularity, venous pattern, temperature, texture, turgor, elasticity, moisture, Lesions.
- ➤ **CAROTID PULSE** - palpate (one at a time) noting amplitude (grade) & equality (symmetry). Auscultate noting absence of bruits.
- ➤ **JVP** (JUGULAR VENOUS PRESSURE) – assess vertical height from sternal angle, with patient supine at 30-45 degrees.
- ➤ **RADIAL PULSE** - palpate noting amplitude and equality
- ➤ **INSPECT & PALPATE LOWER LIMBS** – for swelling, oedema, tenderness, colour, vascularity, varicosities, temperature, venous pattern, pigmentation, hair distribution, texture, turgor, elasticity, moisture,
- ➤ **FEMORAL PULSE** - palpate noting amplitude and equality. Auscultate noting absence of bruits

- ➢ **POPLITEAL** - palpate noting amplitude and equality
- ➢ **POSTERIOR TIBIAL** - palpate noting amplitude and equality
- ➢ **DORSALIS PEDIS** - palpate noting amplitude and equality

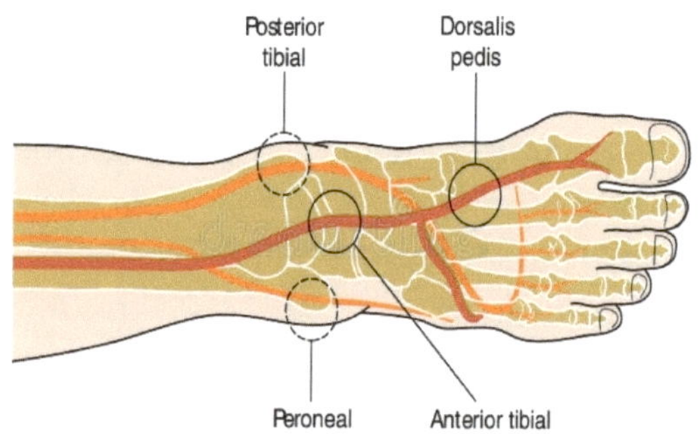

MUSCULOSKELETAL

NECK

- ➤ **INSPECT & PALPATE** - for size, shape, symmetry
- ➤ **ROM** – note range of motion through flexion, extension, rotation, and lateral bending.
- ➤ **STRENGTH** - assess turning face and shrug against resistance (CN XI Spinal Accessory).

BACK

- ➤ **INSPECT** – posture and profile (from side, behind and on bending) noting symmetry and absence of curves, deformities, swelling, redness (msk) noting body position, muscle bulk & tone, involuntary movements (neuro).
- ➤ **PALPATE** – vertebrae and surrounding musculature noting absence of tenderness, deformities, swelling, heat.
- ➤ **ROM** - stabilise pelvis and assess range of motion through flexion, extension, rotation, and lateral bending. Note symmetry. Passive straight leg raise test, dorsiflexion.

The Spine

C1
Cervical vertebrae
C7
T1
C4 injury (quadriplegia)
C6 injury (quadriplegia)
Thoracic vertebrae
T6 injury (paraplegia)
L1 injury (paraplegia)
T12
L1
Lumbar vertebrae
L5
S1
Sacrum & coccyx
S5

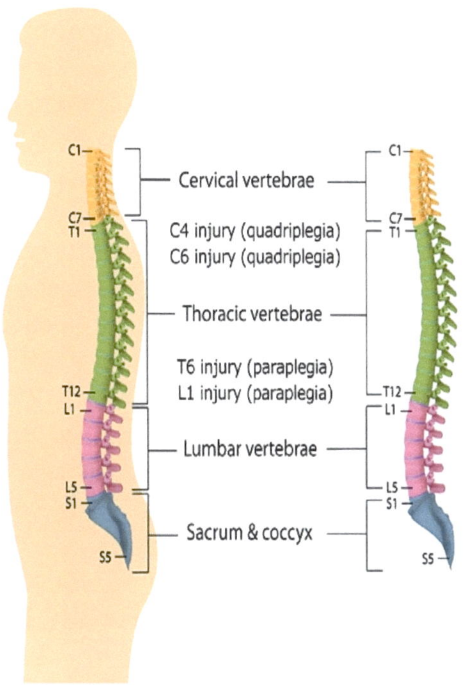

UPPER LIMBS

- ➢ **INSPECT & PALPATE** – noting symmetry, absence of deformities, atrophy, redness, swelling, tenderness, crepitus MSK body position, muscle bulk, tone & involuntary movements (neuro)
- ➢ **ROM** – note range of motion, for: **Shoulders** (abduction, adduction, internal rotation, external rotation, signs of instability-resisted abduction & medial & lateral rotation); **Elbows** (flexion, extension, pronation, supination); **Wrists** (flexion, extension, ulna deviation, radial deviation); **Fingers** including PIP and DIP joints (flexion, extension, abduction, adduction, opposition of thumb).
- ➢ **UPPER LIMB STRENGTH** – assess range of movements against resistance for **Elbows** (flexion, extension), **Wrists** (extension), **Hands** (grip), and **Fingers** (abduction, opposition of thumb).

LOWER LIMBS

- ➢ **INSPECT & PALPATE** – noting symmetry, absence of deformities, atrophy, redness, swelling, tenderness, crepitus (MSK) body position, muscle bulk, tone & involuntary movements (neuro).
- ➢ **ROM** – note range of motion, active if possible, for: **Hips** (flexion, extension, abduction, adduction, internal rotation, external rotation); **Knees** (flexion, extension, signs of instability Valgus MCL stress test, Anterior drawer test-ACL); **Ankles** (dorsiflexion, plantar-flexion, inversion, eversion); **Toes** (flexion, extension).
- ➢ **LOWER LIMB STRENGTH** assess ROM against resistance for **Hips**(flexion, adduction, abduction, extension) **Knees** (extension, flexion), **Ankles** (dorsi & plantar flexion)

COORDINATION

- ➤ **GENERAL & GAIT** - assess as client walks away from and towards examiner, tandem walk and walking on toes then heels, hop on alternate legs and shallow knee bends.
- ➤ **ROMBERG TEST** - note stability (protect from falling)
- ➤ **RAPID ALTERNATING MOVEMENTS** of hands and feet
- ➤ **POINT-TO-POINT** - finger to examiner's finger then client's nose (or chin) several times and heel to knee then down shin to ankle on both sides, bilaterally.

SENSORY

- ➢ **LIGHT** - elicit feelings of light touch using wisp of cotton 3 places (3 branches of CN V Trigeminal nerve) on both sides of face, 2 places on both sides of trunk, and 2 on each extremity
- ➢ **PIN** - elicit feelings of superficial pain (using pin point to stimulate sharp sensation and rounded pin area to stimulate dull sensation for control) 3 places on both sides of face (CN V), 2 places on both sides of trunk, and 2 on each extremity
- ➢ **VIBRATION** – use 128Hz tuning fork to elicit responses to vibrations at distal joints of hands and feet.
- ➢ **POSITION SENSE** - holding at sides, move a finger and big toe to elicit position sense as up or down, bilaterally.
- ➢ **DISCRIMINATION** - assess using stereognosis (ability to identify a small object placed in one hand at a time).

REFLEXES

Assess using reflex hammer noting symmetry and grading on a 0-4+ scale with 2+ being average. Use reinforcement (augmentation) if necessary.

- ➤ **BRACHIAL** - brachioradialis (2.5 - 5cm above wrist)
- ➤ **BICEPS** - using indirect technique in antecubital space
- ➤ **TRICEPS** - with arm across body or supported by examiner with lower arm dangling while striking above elbow
- ➤ **PATELLAR** – at insertion of patellar tendon
- ➤ **ACHILLES** - apply slight stretch by lifting foot to 90 degree angle then strike tendon above heel
- ➤ **PLANTAR RESPONSE** - using end of reflex hammer, stroke from heel to sole along lateral side of foot continuing across under toes to big toe to elicit toe flexion (Babinski response indicated by dorsiflexion of big toe and fanning)

KNEE

Femur
(thighbone)
Anterior cruciate
ligament (ACL)
Medial collatera
ligament (MCL)
Patellar
ligament
Articular
cartilage
Posterior cruciate
ligament (PCL)
Lateral
Meniscus
Medial
Meniscus
Blood
vessels
Tibia
(shinbone)
Fibula

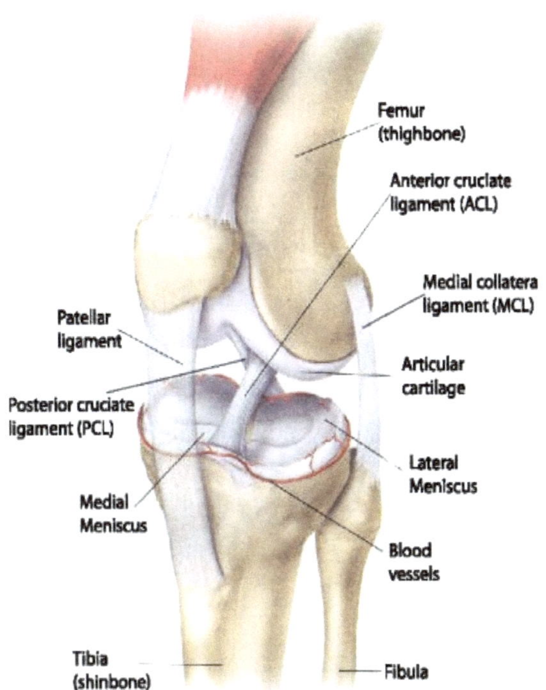

Inspection:

- Exposure- knees, pelvis, lower legs, compare
- Walking, standing, sitting, supine, is pelvis level? Knees symmetrical, anteria / posterior, leg lengths equal.
- Swelling, erythema, scars/wounds.

Palpation: anterior / posterior / lateral

- Patella/patellar ligament/prepatellar bursae.
- Quadriceps, Effusions
- Medial/lateral femoral epicondyles
- Medial/lateral menisci, MCL/LCL
- Biceps femoris (handstring),
- Gastrocnemius / semimembranous bursae
- Popliteal fossa-nodes/artery
- Semimembranous muscle

Movement:

- Flexion, Extension / hyperextension
- Straight leg raising, Resistance flexion
- Resistance extension

- Test I: valgus stress test

  1. Assess integrity of MCL, Pt supine & test knee   extension & flexed 15-20 degrees.
  2. Push knee medially with one hand whilst applying an opposing lateral force at ankle with other hand.
  3. Extension – MNC instability feel separation of tibia & femur & laxity (major disruption).
  4. Flexion – isolates MCL, looking for increased laxity.

- Test II: anterior drawer rest

  1. For ACL, patient supine knee flexed 90 degree.
  2. Grasp tibia just below joint line & pull forward with   both hands.
  3. Intact ACL moves only a few mm & stops abruptly.
  4. Injured ACL has forward movement & a soft end point.

- Test III: Apley / Grinding test

1. Is joint line pain meniscal or ligamentous?
2. Patient prone, knee flexed 90 degree, external / internal rotation, downward force – pain indicates meniscal damage.
3. Repeat external / internal rotation, upward force – pain indicates ligamentous damage

Shoulder

Humerus virtually dangles from scapula, suspended from glenoid fossa by joint capsula, intra-articular capsular ligaments, glenoid labrum, muscles, & tendons.
scapula is anchored to axial skeleton only by sternoclavicular joint & inserting muscles = **scapulothoracic articulation**

3 points orient you to anatomy of shoulder: tip of acromion, greater tubercle of humerus, coracoid process

3 joints articulate at shoulder:

> **glenohumeral joint** (head of humerus with glenoid fossa (not normally palpable)
> **sternoclavicular joint**
> **acromioclavicular joint** (pain is top of shoulder, radiating toward neck)

scapulohumeral group (SITS muscles – rotator cuff): supraspinatus, infraspinatus & teres minor, subscapularis (pain is lateral part of shoulder, radiating toward deltoid insertion) subscapularis is the only one in this group that is not palpable

axioscapular group: trapezius, rhomboids, serratus anterior, levator scapulae

axiohumeral group: pectoralis major & minor, latissimus dorsi

Testing muscles: supraspinatus (pt abducts against resistance), subscapularis (pt rotates forearm medially against resistance), infraspinatus & teres minor (pt rotates forearm laterally against resistance), **thoracohumeral** group (pt adducts forearm against resistance)

- **articular capsule** is lined by a synovial membrane with two outpouchings – the subscapular bursa & the synovial sheath of the tendon of the long head of biceps.
- **biceps tendon** we palpate is from the long head of the biceps; lies in **bicipital groove** between greater & lesser tubercles (pain is anterior shoulder)
- **subacromial bursa** is principal bursa of the shoulder – between acromion & head of humerus
- **subacromial bursitis** – tenderness just below tip of acromion, pain with abduction & rotation

A Normal Shoulder

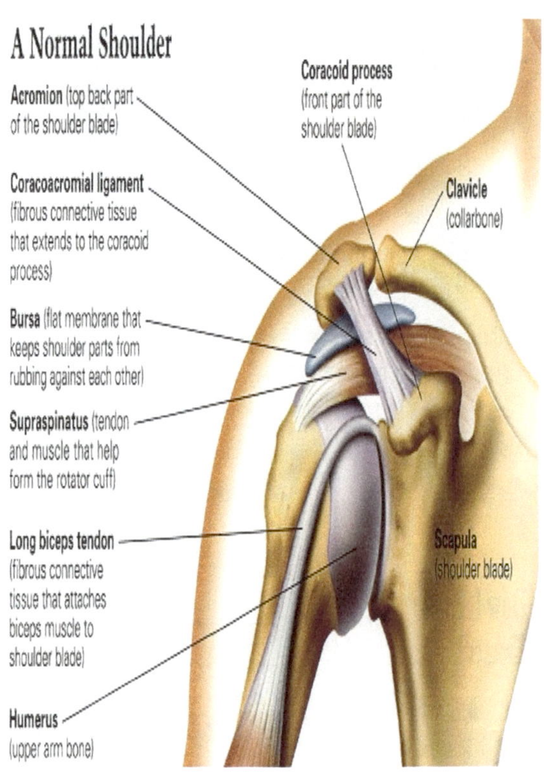

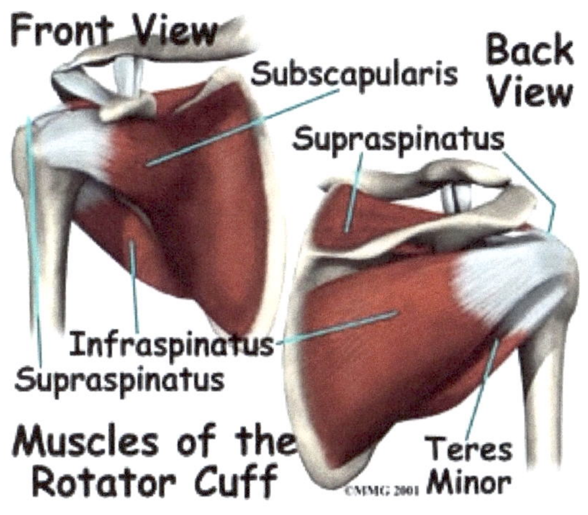

Front View
Subscapularis
Back View
Supraspinatus
Infraspinatus
Supraspinatus
Teres Minor
Muscles of the Rotator Cuff
©MMG 2001

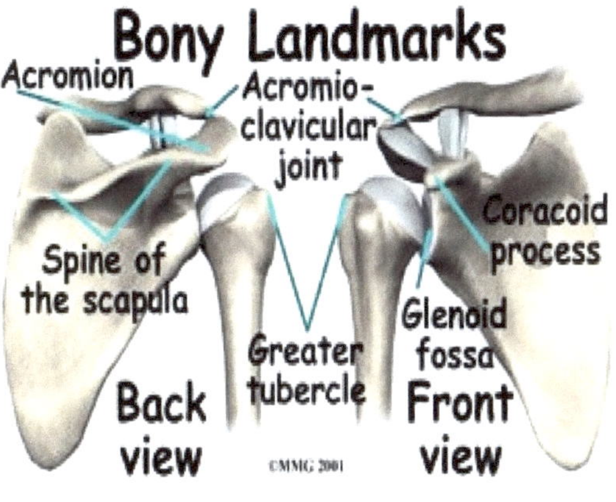

Bony Landmarks
Acromion
Acromio-clavicular joint
Coracoid process
Spine of the scapula
Greater tubercle
Glenoid fossa
Back view
Front view
©MMG 2001

Useful websites

http://emc.medicines.org.uk/

http://medinfo.ufl.edu/year1/bcs/index.html

http://www.bnf.org/bnf/

http://www.practitionersassoc.co.uk

http://www.kingsfund.org.uk/index.html

http://www.library.nhs.uk/Default.aspx

http://www.nice.org.uk/

http://www.npc.co.uk/

http://www.patient.co.uk/patientplus.asp

http://www.pjonline.com/Index.html

http://www.sign.ac.uk/